C000155668

The Definitive KETO Chaffle Cookbook

Delicious Chaffle Recipes To Boost Weight Loss

Rory Kemp

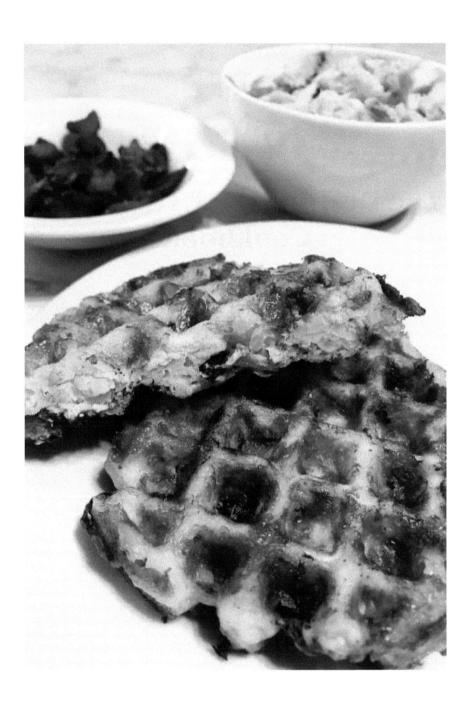

© Copyright 2020 - All rights reserved.

The content contained within this book may not be reproduced, duplicated or transmitted without direct written permission from the author or the publisher.

Under no circumstances will any blame or legal responsibility be held against the publisher, or author, for any damages, reparation, or monetary loss due to the information contained within this book. Either directly or indirectly.

Legal Notice:

This book is copyright protected. This book is only for personal use. You cannot amend, distribute, sell, use, quote or paraphrase any part, or the content within this book, without the consent of the author or publisher.

Disclaimer Notice:

Please note the information contained within this document is for educational and entertainment purposes only. All effort has been executed to present accurate, up to date, and reliable, complete information. No warranties of any kind are declared or implied. Readers acknowledge that the author is not engaging in the rendering of legal, financial, medical or professional advice. The content within this book has been derived from various sources. Please consult a licensed professional before attempting any techniques outlined in this book.

By reading this document, the reader agrees that under no circumstances is the author responsible for any losses, direct or indirect, which are incurred as a result of the use of information contained within this document, including, but not limited to, — errors, omissions, or inaccuracies.

Table of contents

5

Crispy Crab Chaffle

Preparation: 25 minutes

Cooking: 10 minutes

Servings: 2

Ingredients

For chaffle:

- Egg: 1
- Mozzarella cheese: ½ cup (shredded)
- Salt: ¼ tsp or as per your taste
- Black pepper: ¼ tsp or as per your taste
- Ginger powder: 1 tbsp

For crab:

- Crab meat: 1 cup
- Butter: 2 tbsp
- Salt: ¼ tsp or as per your taste
- Black pepper: ¼ tsp or as per your taste
- Red chili flakes: ½ tsp

Directions

1. In a frying pan, Melt now butter and fry crab meat for two minutes
2. Add the spices at the end and set aside
3. Mix all the chaffle ingredients well together
4. Pour a thin layer on a Preheat nowed waffle iron
5. Add prepared crab and pour again more mixture over the top
6. Cook the chaffle for around 5 minutes
7. Make as many chaffles as your mixture and waffle maker allow

Crunchy Pickle Chaffles

Preparation: 5 min

Cooking: 5 min

Servings: 2

Ingredients

- Mozzarella– ½ cup
- Eggs – 1
- Pork Panko bread crumbs – ½ cup
- Pickle juice – 1 tbspn
- Pickle slices – 8

Directions

1. Pre-heat waffle iron
2. Mix ingredients and pour thin layer onto waffle iron
3. Add drained pickle slices
4. Top with remaining mixture and cooking till crisp

Nutrition:

Calories 250, Fat 14, Carbs 25, Protein 5

Stuffed Chaffles

Preparation: 15 minutes

Cooking: 15 minutes

Servings: 6

Ingredients

- 1 tbspn extra-virgin olive oil
- 1/4 cup chopped onion
- ½ cup chopped celery
- ¾ teaspn salt ½ teaspn freshly ground black pepper
- ½ teaspn poultry seasoning
- ¼ teaspn dried sage
- 6 cups low-carb dry bread cubes (about ½-inch square)
- ½ cup unsalted butter, Melt nowed
- 1 cup low-sodium chicken broth
- 1 cup cheese
- 4 eggs (separated)

Directions

1. Put the bread cubes in a bowl preferably big size.

2. Mix butter, cheese, egg white and chicken broth together in a bowl
3. In another bowl, mix all vegetables
4. Pour the butter mixture over the bread.
5. Add the vegetable mixture and stir.
6. Leave the stuffing mixture to sit for 5 minutes to completely absorb the liquid, stir it once or twice.
7. Preheat now the waffle iron on medium heat.
8. Lightly grease the waffle iron.
9. Put close to 1/2 cup of the stuffing mix on one section of the waffle iron.
10. Use enough of the mixture to slightly overstuff each section of the waffle iron.
11. Close the lid and press down to compress the stuffing.
12. Bake till golden brown and cohesive.
13. Repeat the baking procedure until all stuffing mixtures are baked.
14. Keep completed stuffles warm
15. Serve cool

Broccoli & Cheese Chaffle

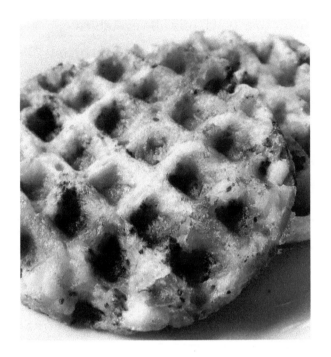

Preparation: 5 minutes

Cooking: 8 minutes

Servings: 2

Ingredients

- ¼ cup broccoli florets
- 1 egg, beaten

- 1 tbspn almond flour
- ¼ teaspn garlic powder
- ½ cup cheddar cheese

Directions

1. Preheat now your waffle maker.
2. Add the broccoli to the food processor.
3. Pulse until chopped.
4. Add to a bowl.
5. Stir in the egg and the rest of the ingredients.
6. Mix well.
7. Pour half of the batter to your waffle maker.
8. Cover and cook for 4 minutes.
9. Repeat procedure to make the next chaffle.

Chaffle with Sausage Gravy

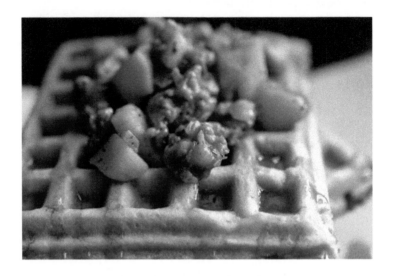

Preparation: 5 minutes

Cooking: 15 minutes

Servings: 2

Ingredients

- ¼ cup sausage, cooked
- 3 tbsps chicken broth
- 2 teaspns cream cheese
- 2 tbsps heavy whipping cream
- ¼ teaspn garlic powder

- Pepper to taste
- 2 basic chaffles (Choose 1 Recipe from Chapter 1)

Directions

1. Add the sausage, broth, cream cheese, cream, garlic powder and pepper to a pan over medium heat.
2. Bring to a boil and then reduce heat.
3. Simmer for 10 minutes or until the sauce has thickened.
4. Pour the gravy on top of the basic chaffles
5. Serve.

Rosemary Pork Chops in Chaffles

Preparation: 10 minutes

Cooking: 15 Minutes

Servings: 2

Ingredients

- 4 eggs
- 2 cups grated mozzarella cheese
- Salt and pepper to taste
- Pinch of nutmeg
- 2 tbsps sour cream
- 6 tbsps almond flour
- 2 teaspns baking powder

Pork chops:

- 2 tbsps olive oil
- 1 pound pork chops
- Salt and pepper to taste
- 1 teaspn freshly chopped rosemary

Other:

- 2 tbsps cooking spray to brush your waffle maker

16

- 2 tbsps freshly chopped basil for decoration

Directions

1. Preheat now your waffle maker.
2. Add the eggs, mozzarella cheese, salt and pepper, nutmeg, sour cream, almond flour and baking powder to a bowl.
3. Mix well until combined.
4. Brush the heated waffle maker with cooking spray and add a few tbsps of the batter.
5. Close the lid and cook for about 7 minutes depending on your waffle maker.
6. Meanwhile, heat the butter in a nonstick grill pan and season the pork chops with salt and pepper and freshly chopped rosemary.
7. Cook the pork chops for about 4–5 minutes on each side.
8. Serve each chaffle with a pork chop and sprinkle some freshly chopped basil on top.

Nutrition:

Calories 666, fat 55.2 g, carbs 4.8 g, sugar 0.4 g, Protein 37.5 g, sodium 235 mg

Spicy Jalapeno Popper Chaffles

Preparation: 10 mins

Cooking: 10 mins

Servings: 1

Ingredients

Chaffle:

- 1 egg
- 1 oz cream cheese, softened
- 1 cup cheddar cheese, shredded

For the toppings:

- 2 tbsp bacon bits
- 1/2 tbsp jalapenos

Directions

1. Turn on your waffle maker. Preheat now for up to 5 minutes.
2. Mix now the chaffle Ingredients.
3. Pour the batter onto your waffle maker.
4. Cook the batter for 3-4 minutes until it's brown and crispy.

5. Remove now the chaffle and repeat steps until all remaining batter have been used up.
6. Sprinkle bacon bits and a few jalapeno slices as toppings.

Nutrition:

calories: 231, carbohydrate: 2g, fat: 18g, protein: 13g

Eggnog Chaffles

Preparation: 15 minutes

Cooking: 10 minutes

Servings: 1

Ingredients

- 1 egg, separated
- 1 egg yolk
- 1/2 cup mozzarella cheese Shredded
- 1/2 tsp spiced rum
- 1 tsp vanilla extract
- 1/4 tsp nutmeg, dried
- A dash of cinnamon
- 1 tsp coconut flour

For the icing:

- 2 tbsp cream cheese
- 1 tbsp powdered sweetener
- 2 tsp rum or rum extract

Directions

1. Preheat now the mini waffle maker.

2. Mix egg yolk in a tiny bowl until smooth.
3. Add in the sweetener and Mix well until the powder is completely dissolved.
4. Add the coconut flour, cinnamon, and nutmeg. Mix well.
5. In another bowl, mix rum, egg white, and vanilla. Whisk until well combined.
6. Throw in the yolk mixture with the egg white mixture. You should be able to form a thin batter.
7. Add the mozzarella cheese and combine with the mixture.
8. Separate the batter into two batches. Put 1/2 of the batter into your waffle maker and let it cook for 6 minutes until it's solid.
9. Repeat until you've used up the remaining batter.
10. In a separate bowl, mix all the icing Ingredients.
11. Top the cooked chaffles with the icing or use it as a dip.

Nutrition:

calories: 266, carbohydrates: 2g, fat: 23g, protein: 13g

Cheddar Jalapeno Chaffles

Preparation: 15 minutes

Cooking: 10 minutes

Servings: 1

Ingredients

- 1 egg
- 1/2 cup cheddar cheese shredded
- 1 tbsp almond flour
- 1 tbsp jalapenos
- 1 tbsp olive oil

Directions

1. Preheat now your waffle maker.
2. While waiting for your waffle maker to heat up, mix jalapeno, egg, cheese, and almond flour in a tiny mixing bowl.
3. Lightly grease your waffle maker with olive oil.
4. In the center of your waffle maker, carefully pour the chaffle batter. Spread the mixture evenly toward the edges.

5. Close your waffle maker lid and wait for 3-4 minutes for the mixture to cook. For an even crispier texture, wait for another 1-2 minutes.
6. Remove now the chaffle. Let it cool before serving.

Nutrition:

calories: 509, carbohydrates: 5g, fat: 45g, protein: 23g

Spicy Jalapeno & Bacon Chaffles

Cooking: 5 Minutes

Servings: 2

Ingredients

- 1 oz. cream cheese
- 1 large egg
- 1/2 cup cheddar cheese
- 2 tbsps. bacon bits
- 1/2 tbsp. jalapenos
- 1/4 tsp baking powder

Directions

1. Switch on your waffle maker.
2. Grease your waffle maker with cooking spray and let it heat up.
3. Mix egg and vanilla extract in a bowl first.
4. Add baking powder, jalapenos and bacon bites.
5. Add in cheese last and mix.

6. Pour the chaffles batter into the maker and cook the chaffles for about 2-3 minutes. Once chaffles are cooked, Remove now from the maker.
7. Serve hot and enjoy!

Nutrition:

Protein: 24% 5kcal, Fat: 70% 175 kcal, Carbohydrates: 6% 15 kcal

Zucchini Parmesan Chaffles

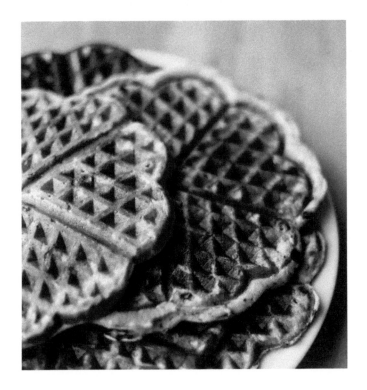

Cooking: 14 Minutes

Servings: 2

Ingredients

- 1 cup shredded zucchini
- 1 egg, beaten
- ½ cup finely grated Parmesan cheese

- Salt and freshly ground black pepper to taste

Directions

1. Preheat now the waffle iron.
2. Put all the ingredients in a bowl and mix well.
3. Open the iron and add half of the mixture.
4. Close and cook until crispy, 7 minutes.
5. Remove now the chaffle onto a plate and make another with the remaining mixture.
6. Cut each chaffle into wedges and serve afterward.

Nutrition:

Calories 138, Fats 9.07g, Carbs 3.81g, Net Carbs 3.71g, Protein 10.02g

Cheeseburger Chaffle

Cooking: 15 Minutes

Servings: 2

Ingredients

- 1 lb. ground beef
- 1 onion, minced
- 1 tsp. parsley, chopped
- 1 egg, beaten
- Salt and pepper to taste
- 1 tbspn olive oil
- 4 basic chaffles (Choose 1 Recipe From Chapter 1)
- 2 lettuce leaves
- 2 cheese slices
- 1 tbspn dill pickles
- Ketchup
- Mayonnaise

Directions

1. In a large bowl, combine the ground beef, onion, parsley, egg, salt and pepper.

2. Mix well. Form 2 thick patties.

3. Add olive oil to the pan. Place the pan over medium heat.

4. Cook the patty for 3 to 5 minutes per side or until fully cooked.

5. Place the patty on top of each chaffle.

6. Top with lettuce, cheese and pickles.

7. Squirt ketchup and mayo over the patty and veggies.

8. Top with another chaffle.

Nutrition:

Calories 325, Total Fat 16.3g, Saturated Fat 6.5g, Cholesterol 157mg, Sodium 208mg, Total Carbohydrate 3g, Dietary Fiber 0.7g, Total Sugars 1.4g, Protein 39.6g, Potassium 532mg

Scallion Cream Cheese Chaffle

Preparation: 6 minutes

Cooking: 20 Minutes

Servings: 2

Ingredients

- 1 large egg
- ½ cup of shredded mozzarella
- 2 Tbsp cream cheese
- 1 Tbsp everything bagel seasoning
- 1-2 sliced scallions

Directions

1. Turn on waffle maker to heat and oil it with cooking spray.
2. Beat egg in a tiny bowl.
3. Add in ½ cup mozzarella.
4. Pour half of the mixture into your waffle maker and cook for 3-minutes.
5. Remove now chaffle and Repeat now with remaining mixture.

30

6. Let them cool, then cover each chaffle with cream cheese, sprinkle with seasoning and scallions.

Nutrition:

Calories 40, Fat 2.2, Fiber 1.8, Carbs 4.3, Protein 1.1

Chicken Taco Chaffles

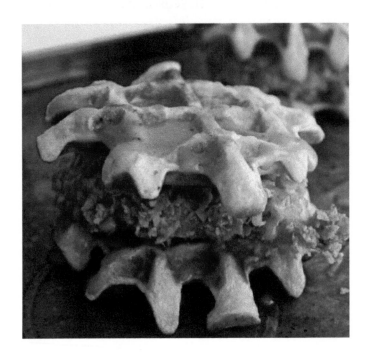

Preparation: 6 minutes

Cooking: 8 Minutes

Servings: 2

Ingredients

- 1/3 cup of cooked grass-fed chicken, chopped
- 1 organic egg

- 1/3 cup of Monterrey Jack cheese, shredded
- ¼ teaspn taco seasoning

Directions

1. Preheat now a mini waffle iron and then grease it.
2. In a bowl, place all the ingredients and Mix well until well combined.
3. Place half of the mixture into Preheat nowed waffle iron and cook for about 4 minutes or until golden brown.
4. Repeat now with the remaining mixture.
5. Serve warm.

Nutrition:

Calories 257, Fat 15.9, Fiber 4.5, Carbs 10.5, Protein 21.5

Cauliflower Turkey Chaffle

Preparation: 6 minutes

Cooking: 12 Minutes

Servings: 2

Ingredients

- 1 large egg (beaten)
- ½ cup cauliflower rice
- ¼ cup diced turkey
- ½ tsp. coconut aminos or soy sauce
- A pinch of ground black pepper
- A pinch of white pepper
- ¼ tsp. curry
- ¼ tsp. oregano
- 1 tbsp. butter (Melt nowed)
- ¾ cup shredded Mozzarella cheese
- 1 garlic clove (crushed)

Directions

1. Plug your waffle maker to Preheat now it and spray it with a non-stick spray.
2. In a mixing bowl, combine the cauliflower rice, white pepper, black pepper, curry and oregano.
3. In another mixing bowl, whisk together the eggs, butter, crushed garlic and coconut aminos.
4. Pour the egg mixture into the cheese mixture and Mix well until the ingredients are well combined.
5. Add the diced turkey and stir to combine.
6. Sprinkle 2 tbsp. cheese over your waffle maker. Fill your waffle maker with an appropriate amount of the batter. Spread out the batter to the edges to cover all the holes on your waffle maker. Sprinkle another 2-tbsp. cheese over the batter.
7. Close your waffle maker and cooking for about 4 minutes or according to waffle maker's settings.
8. After the cooking cycle, use a plastic or silicone utensil to Remove now the chaffle from your waffle maker.
9. Repeat step 6 to 8 until you have cooked all the batter into chaffles.
10. Serve warm and enjoy.

Nutrition:

Calories 112, Fat 8.7, Fiber 0.7, Carbs 2.8, Protein 6.7

Pumpkin Spice Chaffles

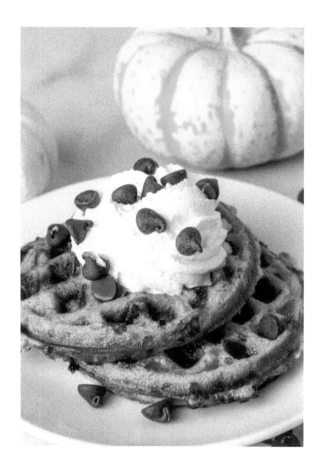

Preparation: 30 minutes

Cooking: 14 Minutes

Servings: 2

Ingredients

- 1 egg, beaten
- ½ tsp. pumpkin pie spice
- ½ cup finely grated Mozzarella cheese
- 1 tbsp. sugar-free pumpkin puree

Directions

1. Preheat now the waffle iron.
2. In a bowl, mix all the ingredients.
3. Open the iron, pour in half of the batter, close, and cooking until crispy, 6 to 7 minutes.
4. Remove now the chaffle onto a plate and set aside.
5. Make another chaffle with the remaining batter.
6. Allow cooling and serve afterward.

Nutrition:

Kcal 468, Fat 38g, Net Carbs 2g, Protein 26g

Open-faced Ham & Green Bell Pepper Chaffle Sandwich

Preparation: 20 minutes

Cooking: 10 Minutes

Servings: 2

Ingredients

- 2 slices ham
- Cooking spray
- 1 green bell pepper, sliced into strips
- 2 slices cheese
- 1 tbspn black olives, pitted and sliced
- 2 basic chaffles (Choose 1 Recipe from Chapter 1)

Directions

1. Cooking the ham in a pan coated with oil over medium heat.
2. Next, cooking the bell pepper.
3. Assemble the open-faced sandwich by topping each chaffle with ham and cheese, bell pepper and olives.

4. Toast in the oven until the cheese has Melt nowed a little.

Nutrition:

Kcal 340, Fat 30.2g, Net Carbs 3.1g, Protein 15g

Mozzarella Peanut Chaffle

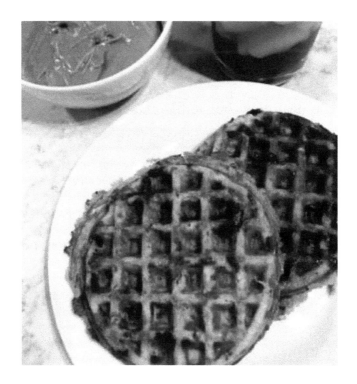

Preparation: 20 minutes

Cooking: 15 Minutes

Servings: 2

Ingredients

- 1 egg, lightly beaten
- 2 tbsp. peanut butter

- 2 tbsp. Swerve
- 1/2 cup Mozzarella cheese, shredded

Directions

1. Preheat now your waffle maker.
2. In a bowl, mix egg, cheese, Swerve, and peanut butter until well combined.
3. Spray waffle maker with cooking spray.
4. Pour half batter in the hot waffle maker and cooking for minutes or until golden brown. Repeat now with the remaining batter.
5. Serve and enjoy.

Nutrition:

Kcal 515, Fat 34.2g, Net Carbs 7.3g, Protein 50.8g

Cinnamon and Vanilla Chaffle

Preparation: 10 minutes

Cooking: 7–9 Minutes

Servings: 4

Ingredients

<u>Batter:</u>

- 4 eggs
- 4 ounce ofs sour cream
- 1 teaspn vanilla extract
- 1 teaspn cinnamon
- ¼ cup stevia
- 5 tbsps coconut flour

<u>Other:</u>

- 2 tbsps coconut oil to brush your waffle maker
- ½ teaspn cinnamon for garnishing the chaffles

Directions

1. Preheat now your waffle maker.

2. Add the eggs and sour cream to a bowl and stir with a wire whisk until combined.

3. Add the vanilla extract, cinnamon, and stevia and Mix well until combined.

4. Stir in the coconut flour and stir until combined.

5. Brush the heated waffle maker with coconut oil and add a few tbsps of the batter.

6. Close the lid and cooking for about 7–8 minutes depending on your waffle maker.

5. Serve and enjoy.

Nutrition:

Kcal 430, Fat 23g, Net Carbs 3g, Protein 33g

Sausage & Pepperoni Chaffle Sandwich

Preparation: 15 minutes

Cooking: 10 Minutes

Servings: 4

Ingredients

- Cooking spray
- 2 cervelat sausage, sliced into rounds
- 12 pieces pepperoni
- 6 mushroom slices
- 4 teaspns mayonnaise
- 4 big white onion rings
- 4 basic chaffles (Choose 1 Recipe from Chapter 1)

Directions

1. Spray your skillet with oil.
2. Place over medium heat.
3. Cooking the sausage until brown on both sides.
4. Transfer on a plate.
5. Cooking the pepperoni and mushrooms for 2 minutes.

6. Spread mayo on top of the chaffle.

7. Top with the sausage, pepperoni, mushrooms and onion rings.

8. Top with another chaffle.

Nutrition:

Kcal 452, Fat 36.4g, Net Carbs 4g, Protein 24g

Pizza Flavored Chaffle

Preparation: 15 minutes

Cooking: 12 Minutes

Servings: 3

Ingredients

- 1 egg, beaten
- ½ cup cheddar cheese, shredded
- 2 tbsps pepperoni, chopped
- 1 tbspn keto marinara sauce
- 4 tbsps almond flour
- 1 teaspn baking powder
- ½ teaspn dried Italian seasoning
- Parmesan cheese, grated

Directions

1. Preheat now your waffle maker.
2. In a bowl, mix now the egg, cheddar cheese, pepperoni, marinara sauce, almond flour, baking powder and Italian seasoning.
3. Add the mixture to your waffle maker.

4. Close the device and cooking for minutes.

5. Open it and transfer chaffle to a plate.

6. Let cool for 2 minutes.

7. Repeat the steps with the remaining batter.

8. Top with the grated Parmesan and serve.

Nutrition:

Kcal 485, Fat 35g, Net Carbs 2g, Protein 26g

Walnuts Low Carb Chaffles

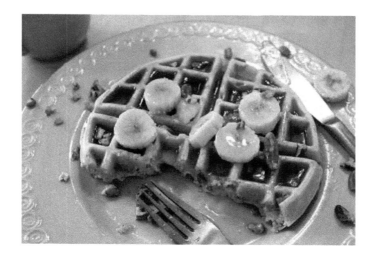

Preparation: 10 minutes

Cooking: 5 minutes

Servings: 2

Ingredients

- 2 tbsps. cream cheese
- ½ tsp. almonds flour
- ¼ tsp. baking powder
- 1 large egg
- ¼ cup chopped walnuts
- Pinch of stevia extract powder

49

Directions

1. Preheat now your waffle maker.

2. Spray waffle maker with cooking spray.

3. In a bowl, add cream cheese, almond flour, baking powder, egg, walnuts, and stevia.

4. Mix all ingredients,

5. Spoon walnut batter in your waffle maker and cooking for about 2-3 minutes.

6. Let chaffles cool at room temperature before serving.

Nutrition:

Kcal 492, Fat: 36g, Net Carbs: 3g, Protein: 35g

Bacon, Egg & Avocado Chaffle Sandwich

Preparation: 15 minutes

Cooking: 10 Minutes

Servings: 2

Ingredients

- Cooking spray
- 4 slices bacon
- 2 eggs
- ½ avocado, mashed
- 4 basic chaffles (Choose 1 from Chapter 1)
- 2 leaves lettuce

Directions

1. Coat your skillet with cooking spray.
2. Cooking the bacon until golden and crisp.
3. Transfer into a paper towel lined plate.
4. Crack the eggs into the same pan and cooking until firm.
5. Flip and cooking until the yolk are set.

6. Spread the avocado on the chaffle.

7. Top with lettuce, egg and bacon.

8. Top with another chaffle.

Nutrition:

Kcal 350, Fat 11g, Net Carbs 3.5g, Protein 34g

Cheddar Chicken and Broccoli Chaffle

Preparation: 2 minutes

Cooking: 8 minutes

Servings: 2

Ingredients

- 1/4 cup cooked diced chicken
- 1/4 cup fresh broccoli chopped
- Shredded Cheddar cheese
- 1 egg
- 1/4 tsp garlic powder

Directions

1. Heat up your waffle maker.
2. In a tiny bowl, mix now the egg, garlic powder, and cheddar cheese.
3. Add the broccoli and chicken and mix well.
4. Add 1/2 of the batter into your mini waffle maker and cook for 4 minutes. If they are still a bit uncooked, leave it cooking for another 2 minutes. Then cook the

rest of the batter to make a second chaffle and then cook the third chaffle.

5. After cooking, Remove now from the pan and let sit for 2 minutes.

6. Dip in ranch dressing, sour cream, or enjoy alone.

Spinach & Artichoke Chicken Chaffle

Preparation: 3 minutes

Cooking: 8 minutes

Servings: 2

Ingredients

- 1/3 cup of cooked diced chicken
- 1/3 cup of cooked spinach chopped
- 1/3 cup of marinated artichokes chopped
- 1/3 cup of shredded mozzarella cheese
- 1 ounce of softened cream cheese
- 1/4 teaspn garlic powder
- 1 egg

Directions

1. Heat up your waffle maker.
2. In a tiny bowl, mix now the egg, garlic powder, cream cheese, and Mozzarella Cheese.
3. Add the spinach, artichoke, and chicken and mix well.

4. Add 1/3 of the batter into your waffle maker and cook for 4 minutes. If they are still a bit uncooked, leave it cooking for another 2 minutes. Then cook the rest of the batter to make a second chaffle and then cook the third chaffle.
5. After cooking, Remove now from the pan and let sit for 2 minutes.
6. Dip in ranch dressing, sour cream, or enjoy alone.

Bacon Chaffles For Couples

Cooking: 5 Minutes

Servings: 2

Ingredients

Chaffle:

- 2 eggs
- 1/2 cup cheddar cheese
- 1/2 cup mozzarella cheese
- 1/4 tsp baking powder
- 1/2 Tbsp almond flour
- 1 Tbsp butter, for waffle maker

For the filling:

- 1/4 cup bacon, chopped
- 2 Tbsp green onions, chopped

Directions

1. Turn on waffle maker to heat and oil it with cooking spray.

2. Add eggs, mozzarella, cheddar, almond flour, and baking powder to a blender and pulse 10 times, so cheese is still chunky.
3. Add bacon and green onions. Pulse 2-times to combine.
4. Add one half of the batter to your waffle maker and cook for 3 min, until golden brown.
5. Repeat now with remaining batter.
6. Add your TOPPINGs and serve hot.

Nutrition:

Carbs: 3 g ;Fat: 3 8 g ;Protein: 23 g ;Calories: 446

Mixed Berries-Vanilla Chaffles

Preparation: 10 minutes

Cooking: 28 minutes

Servings: 4

Ingredients

- 1 egg, beaten
- ½ cup finely grated Mozzarella cheese
- 1 tbsp. cream cheese, softened
- 1 tbsp. sugar-free maple syrup
- 2 strawberries, sliced
- 2 raspberries, slices
- ¼ tsp. blackberry extract
- ¼ tsp. vanilla extract
- ½ cup plain yogurt for serving

Directions

1. Preheat now the waffle iron.
2. In a bowl, mix all the ingredients except the yogurt.
3. Open the iron, lightly grease with cooking spray and pour in a quarter of the mixture.

4. Close the iron and cooking until golden brown and crispy, 7 minutes.

5. Remove now the chaffle onto a plate and set aside.

6. Make three more chaffles with the remaining mixture.

7. To serve: top with the yogurt and enjoy.

Nutrition:

Calories: 99 Cal, Total Fat: 8 g, Saturated Fat: 0 g, Cholesterol: 0 mg, Sodium: 0 mg, Total Carbs: 4 g

Grill Pork Chaffle Sandwich

Cooking: 15 Minutes

Servings: 2

Ingredients

- 1/2 cup mozzarella, shredded
- 1 egg
- I pinch garlic powder

Pork Patty:

- 1/2 cup pork, minutesced
- 1 tbsp. green onion, diced
- 1/2 tsp Italian seasoning
- Lettuce leaves

Directions

1. Preheat now the square waffle maker and grease with
2. Mix egg, cheese and garlic powder in a tiny mixing bowl.
3. Pour batter in a Preheat nowed waffle maker and close the lid.
4. Make 2 chaffles from thisbatter.

61

5. Cook chaffles for about 2-3 minutesutes until cooked through.

6. Meanwhile, mix pork patty ingredients in a bowl and make 1 large patty.

7. Grill pork patty in a Preheat nowed grill for about 3-4 minutesutes per side until cooked through.

8. Arrange pork patty between two chaffles with lettuce leaves. Cut sandwich to make a triangular sandwich.

9. Enjoy!

Nutrition:

Protein: 48% 85 kcal, Fat: 48% 86 kcal, Carbohydrates: 4% 7 kcal

Chaffle & Chicken Lunch Plate

Cooking: 15 Minutes

Servings: 1

Ingredients

Chaffle:

- 1 large egg
- 1/2 cup jack cheese, shredded
- 1 pinch salt

For Serving:

- 1 chicken leg
- salt
- pepper
- 1 tsp. garlic, minutesced
- 1 egg
- 1 tsp avocado oil

Directions

1. Heat your square waffle maker and grease with cooking spray.

2. Pour Chaffle batter intothe skillet and cook for about 3 minutes.
3. Meanwhile, heat oil in a pan, over medium heat.
4. Once the oil is hot, add chicken thigh and garlic then, cook for about 5 minutes. Flip and cook for another 3-4 minutes.
5. Season with salt and pepper and give them a good mix.
6. Transfer cooked thigh to plate.
7. Fry the egg in the same pan for about 1-2 minutes according to your choice.
8. Once chaffles are cooked, serve with fried egg and chicken thigh.
9. Enjoy!

Nutrition:

Protein: 31% 138 kcal, Fat: 66% 292 kcal, Carbohydrates: 2% kcal

Spicy Shrimp and Chaffles

Cooking: 31 Minutes

Servings: 4

Ingredients

For the shrimp:

- 1 tbsp olive oil
- 1 lb jumbo shrimp, peeled and deveined
- 1 tbsp Creole seasoning
- Salt to taste
- 2 tbsp hot sauce
- 3 tbsp butter
- 2 tbsp chopped fresh scallions to garnish

For the chaffles:

- 2 eggs, beaten
- 1 cup finely grated Monterey Jack cheese

Directions

For the shrimp:

1. Heat the olive oil in a medium skillet over medium heat.
2. Season the shrimp with the Creole seasoning and salt. Cook in the oil until pink and opaque on both sides, 2 minutes.
3. Pour in the hot sauce and butter. Mix well until the shrimp is adequately coated in the sauce, 1 minute.
4. Turn the heat off and set aside.

For the chaffles:

1. Preheat now the waffle iron.
2. In a bowl, mix now the eggs and Monterey Jack cheese.
3. Open the iron and add a quarter of the mixture. Close and cook until crispy, 7 minutes.
4. Transfer the chaffle to a plate and make 3 more chaffles in the same manner.
5. Cut the chaffles into quarters and place on a plate.
6. Top with the shrimp and garnish with the scallions.
7. Serve warm.

Nutrition:

Calories 342, Fats 19.75g, Carbs 2.8g, Net Carbs 2.3g, Protein 36.01g

Hearty Chaffle Dough with Jalapeno

Preparation: 10 minutes

Cooking: 5 minutes

Servings: 2

Ingredients

- 3 large eggs
- 2 to 3 jalapenos, cored, one diced, the other cut into strips
- 4 slices of bacon
- 225 g cream cheese
- 115 g grated cheddar cheese
- 3 tbsp. coconut flour
- 1 teaspn Baking powder
- 1/4 tsp. Himalayan salt

Directions

1. Fry the bacon until crispy in a pan. In the meantime, mix now the dry ingredients and beat the cream cheese in a separate bowl until creamy. Heat the chaffle iron and grease it. Whisk the eggs and fold in

half of the cream cheese and cheese, then the dry
ingredients. Finally, fold in the diced jalapenos.

2. Bake the cheese wafers by putting half of the dough
   in the iron, taking out the chaffle after about 5
   minutes and then baking the other half.

3. Serve the chaffles with the rest of the cream cheese,
   the bacon and the remaining jalapenos.

Nutrition:

Calories 137, Fat 7.9, Fiber 2.3, Carbs 5.1, Protein 7.2

Crunchy Fish and Chaffle Bites

Cooking: 15 Minutes

Servings: 4

Ingredients

- 1 lb. cod fillets, sliced into 4 slices
- 1 tsp. sea salt
- 1 tsp. garlic powder
- 1 egg, whisked
- 1 cup almond flour
- 2 tbsp. avocado oil

Chaffle:

- 2 eggs
- 1/2 cup cheddar cheese
- 2 tbsps. almond flour
- ½ tsp. Italian seasoning

Directions:

1. Mix chaffle ingredients in a bowl and make 4 squares
2. Put the chaffles in a Preheat nowed chaffle maker.

3. Mix now the salt, pepper, and garlic powder in a mixing bowl. Toss the cod cubes in this mixture and let sit for 10 minutes.
4. Then dip each cod slice into the egg mixture and then into the almond flour.
5. Heat oil in skillet and fish cubes for about 2-3 min, until cooked and browned
6. Serve on chaffles and enjoy!

Nutrition:

Calories 173, Fat 10.4, Fiber 8.5, Carbs 15.3, Protein 5

Keto Chaffle Stuffing Recipe

Preparation: 5 minutes

Cooking: 12 minutes

Servings: 4

Ingredients

Basic Chaffle:

- 1/2 cup cheese mozzarella, cheddar or a combo of both
- 2 eggs
- 1/4 tsp. garlic powder
- 1/2 tsp. onion powder
- 1/2 tsp. dried poultry seasoning
- 1/4 tsp. salt
- 1/4 tsp. pepper

Stuffing:

- 1 tiny onion diced
- 2 celery stalks
- 4 oz. mushrooms diced
- 4 tbs butter for sauteing
- 3 eggs

Directions

1. First, make your chaffles.

2. Preheat now the mini waffle iron.

3. Preheat now the oven to 350F

4. In a medium-size bowl, combine the chaffle ingredients.

5. Pour a 1/4 of the mixture into a mini waffle maker and cooking each chaffle for about 4 minutes each.

6. Once they are all cooked, set them aside.

7. In a tiny frying pan, sauté the onion, celery, and mushrooms until they are soft.

8. In a separate bowl, tear up the chaffles into tiny pieces, add the sauteed veggies, and 3 eggs. Mix well until the ingredients are fully combined.

9. Add the stuffing mixture to a tiny casserole dish (about a 4 x 4) and bake it at 350 degrees for about 30 to 40 minutes.

Nutrition:

Calories: 298, Fat: 17g, Carbs: 7,2, Protein: 23g.

Chaffle Minutesi Sandwich

Cooking: 10 Minutes

Servings: 2

Ingredients

Chaffle:

- 1 large egg
- 1/8 cup almond flour
- 1/2 tsp. garlic powder
- 3/4 tsp. baking powder
- 1/2 cup shredded cheese

Sandwich Filling:

- 2 slices deli ham
- 2 slices tomatoes
- 1 slice cheddar cheese

Directions

1. Grease your square waffle maker and Preheat now it on medium heat.
2. Mix chaffle ingredients in a mixing bowl until well combined.

3. Pour batter into a square waffle and make two chaffles.

4. Once chaffles are cooked, Remove now from the maker.

5. For a sandwich, arrange deli ham, tomato slice and cheddar cheese between two chaffles.

6. Cut sandwich from the center.

7. Serve and enjoy!

Nutrition:

Protein: 29% 70 kcal, Fat: 66% 159 kcal, Carbohydrates: 4% 10 kcal

Chicken Zinger Chaffle

Cooking: 15 Minutes

Servings: 2

Ingredients

- 1 chicken breast, cut into 2 pieces
- 1/2 cup coconut flour
- 1/4 cup finely grated Parmesan
- 1 tsp. paprika
- 1/2 tsp. garlic powder
- 1/2 tsp. onion powder
- 1 tsp. salt& pepper
- 1 egg beaten
- Avocado oil for frying
- Lettuce leaves
- BBQ sauce

Chaffle:

- 4 oz. cheese
- 2 whole eggs
- 2 oz. almond flour
- 1/4 cup almond flour

- 1 tsp baking powder

Directions

1. Mix chaffle ingredients in a bowl.
2. Pour the chaffle batter in Preheat nowed greased square chaffle maker.
3. Cook chaffles for about 2-minutesutes until cooked through.
4. Make square chaffles from this batter.
5. Meanwhile mix coconut flour, parmesan, paprika, garlic powder, onion powder salt and pepper in a bowl.
6. Dip chicken first in coconut flour mixture then in beaten egg.
7. Heat avocado oil in a skillet and cook chicken from both sides. until lightly brown and cooked
8. Set chicken zinger between two chaffles with lettuce and BBQ sauce.
9. Enjoy!

Nutrition:

Protein: 30% 219 kcal, Fat: 60% 435 kcal, Carbohydrates: 9% 66 kcal

Double Chicken Chaffles

Cooking: 5 Minutes

Servings: 2

Ingredients

- 1/2 cup boil shredded chicken
- 1/4 cup cheddar cheese
- 1/8 cup parmesan cheese
- 1 egg
- 1 tsp. Italian seasoning
- 1/8 tsp. garlic powder
- 1 tsp. cream cheese

Directions

1. Preheat now the waffle maker.
2. Mix the chaffle ingredients in a bowl and mix.
3. Sprinkle 1 tbsp. of cheese in a waffle maker and pour in chaffle batter.
4. Pour 1 tbsp. of cheese over batter and close the lid.
5. Cook chaffles for about 4 to minutes.

6. Serve with a chicken zinger and enjoy the double chicken flavor.

Nutrition:

Protein: 30% 60 kcal, Fat: 65% 129 kcal, Carbohydrates: 5% 9 kcal

Chaffle With Cheese & Bacon

Cooking: 15 Minutes

Servings: 2

Ingredients

- 1 egg
- 1/2 cup cheddar cheese, shredded
- 1 tbsp. parmesan cheese
- 3/4 tsp coconut flour
- 1/4 tsp baking powder
- 1/8 tsp Italian Seasoning
- pinch of salt
- 1/4 tsp garlic powder

For Topping:

- 1 bacon sliced, cooked and chopped
- 1/2 cup mozzarella cheese, shredded
- 1/4 tsp parsley, chopped

Directions

1. Preheat now oven to 400 degrees.

2. Switch on your waffle maker and grease with cooking spray.
3. Mix chaffle ingredients in a mixing bowl until combined.
4. Spoon half of the batter in your waffle maker's center and close the lid. Cook chaffles for about 3-minutesutes until cooked.
5. Carefully Remove now chaffles from the maker.
6. Arrange chaffles in a greased baking tray.
7. Top with mozzarella cheese, chopped bacon and parsley.
8. And bake in the oven for 4 -5 minutes.
9. Once the cheese is Melt nowed, Remove now from the oven.
10. Serve and enjoy!

Nutrition:

Protein: 28% 90 kcal, Fat: 69% 222 kcal, Carbohydrates: 3% kcal

Keto Tuna Melt Chaffle Recipe

Preparation: 15 minutes

Cooking: 8 minutes

Servings: 2

Ingredients

- 1 packet Tuna 2.6 oz. with no water
- 1/2 cup Mozzarella cheese
- 1 egg
- pinch salt

Directions

1. Preheat now the mini waffle maker
2. In a tiny bowl, add the egg and whip it up.
3. Add the tuna, cheese, and salt and mix well.
4. Optional step for an extra crispy crust: Add a teaspn of cheese to the mini waffle maker for about 30 seconds before adding the recipe mixture. This will allow the cheese to get crispy when the tuna chaffle is done cooking. I prefer this method!

5. Add 1/2 the mixture to your waffle maker and cooking it for a minimum of 4 minutes.
6. Remove now it and cooking the last tuna chaffle for another 4 minutes.

Nutrition:

Calories 283, Fat 20.2, Fiber 3.3, Carbs 1.4, Protein 14.5

Blueberry & Brie Grilled Cheese Chaffle

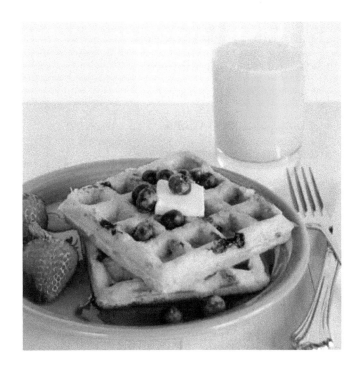

Preparation: 10 minutes

Cooking: 10 minutes

Ingredients

- 2 chaffles
- 1 t blueberry compote
- 1 oz. Wisconsin brie sliced thin
- 1 t Kerry gold butter

Chaffle:

- 1 egg, beaten
- 1/4 cup Mozzarella shredded
- 1 tsp. Swerve confectioners
- 1 T cream cheese softened
- 1/4 tsp. baking powder
- 1/2 tsp. vanilla extract

Blueberry Compote:

- 1 cup blueberries washed
- Zest of 1/2 lemon
- 1 T lemon juice freshly squeezed
- 1 T Swerve Confectioners
- 1/8 tsp. xanthan gum
- 2 T water

Directions

For the Chaffle

1. Mix everything.
2. Cooking 1/2 batter for 2.1/2- 3 minutes in the mini waffle maker
3. Repeat.
4. Let cool slightly on a cooling rack.

For Blueberry Compote

1. Add everything except xanthan gum to a tiny saucepan. Bring to a boil, reduce heat and simmer for 5-10 minutes until it starts to thicken. Sprinkle with xanthan gum and stir well.
2. Remove now from heat and let cool. Store in refrigerator until ready to use.

For Grilled Cheese

1. Heat butter in a tiny pan over medium heat. Place Brie slices on a Chaffle and top with generous 1 T scoop of prepared blueberry compote.
2. Place sandwich in pan and grill, flipping once until waffle is golden and cheese has Melt nowed, about 2 minutes per side.

Nutrition:

Calories 273, Fat 16.7, Fiber 1.5, Carbs 4.1, Protein 11.8

Wasabi Chaffles

Preparation: 15 minutes

Cooking: 15 minutes

Servings: 1

Ingredients

- 1 Basic Chaffle (Choose 1 Recipe from Chapter 1)
- 1 whole avocado, ripe
- 5 slices of pickled ginger
- 1 tbsp. of gluten-free soy sauce
- 1/3 of a cup of edamame
- 1/4 of a cup of Japanese pickled vegetables
- 1/2 pound of sushi-grade salmon, sliced
- 1/4 of a tsp. of wasabi

Directions

1. Cut the salmon and avocado into thin slices. Set aside.
2. If the edamame is frozen, boil it in a pot of water until done. Set aside.
3. Follow the Classic Chaffle recipe.

4. Once the chaffles are done, pour a tbspn of soy sauce onto the chaffle and then layer the salmon, avocado, edamame, pickled ginger, pickled vegetables, and wasabi.
5. Enjoy!

Nutrition:

Calories 321, Fat 14.8, Fiber 4.5, Carbs 6.5, Protein 19.7

Bacon & Serrano Pepper Chaffles

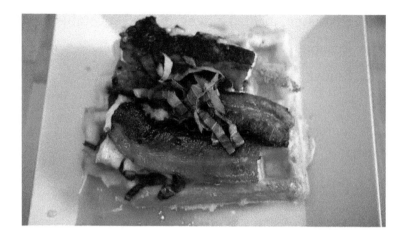

Preparation: 6 minutes

Cooking: 10 Minutes

Servings: 2

Ingredients

- 1 organic egg, beaten
- ½ cup Swiss/Gruyere cheese blend, shredded
- 2 tbsps cooked bacon slices, chopped
- 1 tbspn Serrano pepper, chopped

Directions

1. Preheat now a mini waffle iron and then grease it.
2. In a bowl, place all ingredients and mix well.
3. Place half of the mixture into Preheat nowed waffle iron and cook for about 5 minutes or until golden brown.
4. Repeat now with the remaining mixture.
5. Meanwhile, in a bowl, mix together the cream and stevia for dip.
6. Serve warm.

Nutrition:

Calories 128, Fat 3.2, Fiber 3.9, Carbs 4.9, Protein 4.1

Barbecue Chaffle

Preparation: 5 minutes

Cooking: 8 minutes

Servings: 2

Ingredients

- 1 egg, beaten
- ½ cup cheddar cheese, shredded
- ½ teaspn barbecue sauce
- ¼ teaspn baking powder

Directions

1. Plug in your waffle maker to Preheat now.
2. Mix all the ingredients in a bowl.
3. Pour half of the mixture to your waffle maker.
4. Cover and cook for 4 minutes.
5. Repeat the same steps for the next barbecue chaffle.

Turkey Chaffle Burger

Preparation: 10 minutes

Cooking: 10 minutes

Servings: 2

Ingredients

- 2 cups ground turkey
- Salt and pepper to taste
- 1 tbspn olive oil
- 4 garlic chaffles
- 1 cup Romaine lettuce, chopped
- 1 tomato, sliced
- Mayonnaise
- Ketchup

Directions

1. Combine ground turkey, salt and pepper.
2. Form 2 thick burger patties.
3. Add the olive oil to a pan over medium heat.
4. Cook the turkey burger until fully cooked on both sides.

5. Spread mayo on the chaffle.
6. Top with the turkey burger, lettuce and tomato.
7. Squirt ketchup on top before topping with another chaffle.

Cauliflower Chaffles And Tomatoes

Cooking: 15 Minutes

Servings: 2

Ingredients

- 1/2 cup cauliflower
- 1/4 tsp. garlic powder
- 1/4 tsp. black pepper
- 1/4 tsp. Salt
- 1/2 cup shredded cheddar cheese
- 1 egg

For Topping

- 1 lettuce leave
- 1 tomato sliced
- 4 oz. cauliflower steamed, mashed
- 1 tsp sesame seeds

Directions

1. Add all chaffle ingredients into a blender and mix well.

2. Sprinkle 1/8 shredded cheese on your waffle maker and pour cauliflower mixture in a Preheat nowed waffle maker and sprinkle the rest of the cheese over it.
3. Cook chaffles for about 4-5 minutesutes until cooked
4. For serving, lettuce leaves over chaffle top with steamed cauliflower and tomato.
5. Drizzle sesame seeds on top.
6. Enjoy!

Nutrition:

Protein: 25% 49 kcal, Fat: 65% 128 kcal, Carbohydrates: 10% 21 kcal

Fish and Chaffle Bites

Preparation: 10 minutes

Cooking: 15 minutes

Servings: 2

Ingredients

- 1 lb. cod fillets, sliced into 4 slices
- 1 tsp. sea salt
- 1 tsp. garlic powder
- 1 egg, whisked
- 1 cup almond flour
- 2 tbsp. avocado oil

Chaffle:

- 2 eggs
- 1/2 cup cheddar cheese
- 2 tbsps. almond flour
- ½ tsp. Italian seasoning

Directions

1. Mix chaffle ingredients in a bowl and make 4 squares
2. Put the chaffles in a Preheat nowed chaffle maker.

3. Mix now the salt, pepper, and garlic powder in a mixing bowl. Toss the cod cubes in this mixture and sit for 10 min.

4. Then dip each cod slice into the egg mixture and then into the almond flour.

5. Heat oil in skillet and fish cubes for about 2-3 minutes Utes, until cooked and browned

6. Serve on chaffles and enjoy!

Nutrition:

Protein: 38% 121 kcal, Fat: 59% 189 kcal, Carbohydrates: 3% 11 kcal

Chaffles & Chicken Lunch Plate

Preparation: 10 minutes

Cooking: 15 Minutes

Servings: 2

Ingredients

- 1 large egg
- 1/2 cup jack cheese, shredded
- 1 pinch salt

For Serving:

- 1 chicken leg
- salt
- pepper
- 1 tsp. garlic, minutes
- 1 egg
- 1 tsp avocado oil

Directions

1. Heat your square waffle maker and grease with cooking spray.

2. Pour Chaffle batter into the skillet and cook for about 3 minutes.
3. Meanwhile, heat oil in a pan, over medium heat.
4. Once the oil is hot, add chicken thigh and garlic then, cook for about 5 minutes. Flip and cook for another 3-4 minutes.
5. Season with salt and pepper and give them a good mix.
6. Transfer cooked thigh to plate.
7. Fry the egg in the same pan for about 1-2 minutes Utes according to your choice.
8. Once chaffles are cooked, serve with fried egg and chicken thigh.
9. Enjoy!

Nutrition:

Protein: 31% 138 kcal, Fat: 66% 292 kcal, Carbohydrates: 2% kcal

Crispy Beef Artichoke Chaffle

Preparation: 10 minutes

Cooking: 5 minutes

Servings: 2

Ingredients

- Beef: ½ cup cooked grounded
- Artichokes: 1 cup chopped
- Egg: 1
- Mozzarella cheese: 1/2 cup (shredded)
- Cream cheese: 1 ounce of
- Salt: as per your taste
- Garlic powder: ¼ tsp
- Onion powder: ¼ tsp

Directions

1. Preheat now a mini waffle maker if needed and grease it
2. In a mixing bowl, add all the ingredients
3. Mix now them all well

4. Pour the mixture to the lower plate of your waffle maker and spread it evenly to cover the plate properly

5. Close the lid

6. Cook for at least 4 minutes to get the desired crunch

7. Remove now the chaffle from the heat and keep aside for around one minute

8. Make as many chaffles as your mixture and waffle maker allow

9. Serve hot with your favorite keto sauce

Beef Cheddar Chaffle

Preparation: 15 minutes

Cooking: 8 minutes

Servings: 2

Ingredients

- Beef: 1 cup (grounder)
- Egg: 2
- Chedder cheese: 1 cup
- Mozarrella cheese: 4 tbsp
- Tomato sauce: 6 tbsp
- Basil: ½ tsp
- Garlic: ½ tbsp
- Butter: 1 tsp

Directions

1. In a pan, add butter and include beef
2. Stir for two minutes and then add garlic and basil
3. Cook till tender
4. Set aside the cooked beef
5. Preheat now the mini waffle maker if needed

6. Mix cooked beef, eggs, and 1 cup mozzarella cheese properly
7. Spread it to the mini waffle maker thoroughly
8. Cook for 4 minutes or till it turns crispy and then Remove now it from your waffle maker
9. Make as many mini chaffles as you can
10. Now in a baking tray, line these mini chaffles and top with the tomato sauce and grated mozzarella cheese
11. Put the tray in the oven at 400 degrees until the cheese Melt nows
12. Serve hot with your favorite keto sauce

Beef Broccoli Chaffle

Preparation: 10 minutes

Cooking: 5 minutes

Servings: 2

Ingredients

- Broccoli: ½ cup
- Beef: ½ cup boneless
- Butter: 2 tbsp
- Egg: 1
- Shredded mozzarella: half cup
- Pepper: as per your taste
- Garlic powder: 1 tbsp
- Salt: as per your taste
- Basil: 1 tsp

Directions

1. In a pan, add butter and include beef
2. Stir for two minutes and then add garlic and basil
3. Cook till tender

4. Boil broccoli for 10 minutes in a separate pan and blend
5. Set aside the cooked beef
6. Preheat now the mini waffle maker if needed
7. Mix cooked beef, broccoli blend, eggs, and 1 cup mozzarella cheese properly
8. Spread it to the mini waffle maker thoroughly
9. Cook for 4 minutes or till it turns crispy and then Remove now it from your waffle maker
10. Make as many mini chaffles as you can
11. Now in a baking tray, line these mini chaffles and top with the tomato sauce and grated mozzarella cheese
12. Put the tray in the oven at 400 degrees until the cheese Melt nows
13. Serve hot with your favorite keto sauce

Garlic Lobster Chaffle Roll

Preparation: 5 minutes

Cooking: 5 minutes

Servings: 2

Ingredients

For chaffle:

- Egg: 2
- Mozzarella cheese: 1 cup (shredded)
- Bay seasoning: ½ tsp
- Garlic powder: ¼ tsp

For lobster mix:

- Langostino tails: 1 cup
- Kewpie mayo: 2 tbsp
- Garlic powder: ½ tsp
- Lemon juice: 2 tsp
- Parsley: 1 tsp (chopped) for garnishing

Directions

1. Defrost langostino tails

2. In a tiny mixing bowl, mix langostino tails with lemon juice, garlic powder, and kewpie mayo; mix properly and keep aside

3. In another mixing bowl, beat eggs and add mozzarella cheese to them with garlic powder and bay seasoning

4. Mix now them all well and pour to the greasy mini waffle maker

5. Cook for at least 4 minutes to get the desired crunch

6. Remove now the chaffle from the heat, add the lobster mixture in between and fold

7. Make as many chaffles as your mixture and waffle maker allow

8. Serve hot and enjoy!

Fried Fish Chaffles

Preparation: 15 minutes

Cooking: 10 minutes

Servings: 2

Ingredients

For chaffle:

- Egg: 2
- Mozzarella cheese: 1 cup (shredded)
- Bay seasoning: ½ tsp
- Garlic powder: ¼ tsp

For fried fish:

- Fish boneless: 1 cup
- Garlic powder: 1 tbsp
- Onion powder: 1 tbsp
- Salt: ¼ tsp or as per your taste
- Black pepper: ¼ tsp or as per your taste
- Turmeric: ¼ tsp
- Red chili flakes: ½ tbsp
- Butter: 2 tbsp

Directions

1. Marinate the fish with all the ingredients of the fried fish except for butter
2. Melt now butter in a medium-size frying pan and add the marinated fish
3. Fry from both sides for at least 5 minutes and set aside
4. Preheat now a mini waffle maker if needed and grease it
5. In a mixing bowl, beat eggs and add all the chaffle ingredients
6. Mix now them all well
7. Pour the mixture to the lower plate of your waffle maker and spread it evenly to cover the plate properly
8. Close the lid
9. Cook for at least 4 minutes to get the desired crunch
10. Remove now the chaffle from the heat and keep aside for around one minute
11. Make as many chaffles as your mixture and waffle maker allow
12. Serve hot with the prepared fish

Lightning Source UK Ltd.
Milton Keynes UK
UKHW020635070621
385067UK00001B/28